THE COMPLETE DASH DIET COOKBOOK FOR BEGINNERS 2024

Achieve Lower Blood Pressure Naturally through Simple Healthy Low-Sodium Recipes to Attain Long-Lasting Health

Dr. Raphael Rachelle

TABLE OF CONTENTS

ENCOURAGEMENT

Embarking on the DASH (Dietary Approaches to Stop Hypertension) Diet can be a positive step toward better health and well-being. For beginners setting out on this journey.

Take It One Step at a Time: Starting something new can feel overwhelming, but remember, every small step counts. Take it one day, one meal, and one choice at a time.

Celebrate Progress, Not Perfection: The goal is progress, not perfection. Embrace every small success and effort you make towards a healthier lifestyle.

Change takes time, so be patient and kind to yourself. Be patient with yourself. Give yourself grace and understand that it's okay to have occasional setbacks.

Focus on the Positive Changes: Shift your focus to the positive changes you're making. Whether it's adding more vegetables to your plate or choosing a healthier snack, every choice counts.

Learn and Explore: Use this as an opportunity to learn more about food, nutrition, and your body. Embrace the journey of discovering new, delicious, and healthy foods.

You're Worth It: Your health and well-being matter. Taking steps toward a healthier lifestyle is an investment in yourself and your future.

Support Is Key: Seek support from family, friends, or online communities. Having a support system can make this journey more enjoyable and easier to navigate.

Maintain a Positive Attitude: A positive attitude may go a long way. Celebrate the journey, stay motivated, and focus on the many benefits of living a healthier lifestyle.

You're Not Alone: Many people are on a similar path. Find inspiration and motivation from success stories, and remember, you're not alone in this journey.

You're making a Positive Change: By choosing to embark on the DASH Diet, you're taking a proactive step toward a healthier and happier life.

INTRODUCTION

In the heart of New York City, amidst the bustling streets and towering skyscrapers, a subtle yet profound transformation was underway in the life of Peter, a devoted American citizen determined to reclaim his health. His journey began not in a grand fashion but within the quiet sanctuary of his modest kitchen.

Struggling with the aftermath of a high-stress corporate lifestyle that had taken a toll on his well-being, Peter sought a change. Determined to regain control over his health, he turned to a guiding light—**the "Complete DASH Diet Cookbook for Beginners 2024."** Within the crisp pages of this culinary beacon, he discovered a roadmap to a healthier life, a treasury of flavorful recipes, and a comprehensive guide on embracing the renowned DASH Diet.

Armed with newfound knowledge and an insatiable hunger for change, Peter embarked on a culinary expedition. He shuffled through thc cookbook's pages, uncovering vibrant recipes that sparked his imagination and promised a healthier, more fulfilling way of eating. With measured enthusiasm, he navigated the aisles of his local market, picking out vibrant produce, lean proteins, and wholesome grains as guided by the book's expert advice.

In the confines of his kitchen, culinary alchemy unfolded. Pots and pans simmered with the aroma of freshly prepared meals—colorful salads, succulent grilled fish, and tantalizing vegetable stir-fries, each dish a testament to the transformative power of the DASH Diet. With each sizzle, each savory aroma wafting through the air, Peter felt a newfound sense of purpose and vitality taking root within him.

As days turned into weeks and weeks into months, Peter's energy surged, and the numbers on his blood pressure monitor steadily declined. His journey, inspired and guided by the wisdom nestled in **"The Complete DASH Diet Cookbook for Beginners 2024,"** became a tale of personal triumph. It wasn't just about recipes; it was a narrative of reclaiming health, vitality, and a life brimming with renewed optimism.

In the heart of the metropolis, within the sanctum of his kitchen, Peter discovered the catalyst for his transformation—a cookbook that became a cornerstone in his journey toward a healthier, more vibrant life.

Overview of the DASH Diet principles

The DASH (Dietary Approaches to Stop Hypertension) Diet is a dietary approach aimed at preventing and managing hypertension (high blood pressure) and promoting overall heart health. Its principles revolve around a balanced eating plan that emphasizes whole foods and reduces the intake of sodium, thus contributing to a healthier cardiovascular system.

Fruits and vegetables are emphasized: The DASH Diet supports the eating of a range of fruits and vegetables. These are rich in essential vitamins, minerals, and antioxidants and are naturally low in fat.

Whole Grains: Whole grains are a primary component of the DASH Diet. They provide fiber, essential nutrients, and energy while contributing to better heart health.

Lean Protein Sources: The diet incorporates lean protein sources like poultry, fish, nuts, seeds, and legumes. These options are lower in saturated fats and provide important nutrients.

Low-Fat Dairy Products: The DASH Diet includes dairy products that are low-fat or fat-free. These are important sources of calcium and other nutrients without the saturated fat content found in full-fat dairy.

Limited Saturated Fats and Red Meat: Reducing the consumption of saturated fats and red meat is a cornerstone of the DASH Diet, as these have been linked to an increased Heart disease and excessive blood pressure are both risks.

Reduced Sodium Intake: The DASH Diet emphasizes reducing salt intake. It recommends limiting high-sodium foods and promotes the use of herbs and spices for flavor instead of salt.

Moderation in Added Sugars: The diet advises moderation in the intake of added sugars and sugary beverages to maintain overall health and support healthy weight management.

Balanced Portions and Moderation: Portion control and balanced eating are essential components of the DASH Diet. It promotes a balanced intake of different food groups to ensure a well-rounded diet.

Key advantages and health benefits associated with the DASH Diet

Blood Pressure Management: The primary aim of the DASH Diet is to control and lower blood pressure. It's been clinically proven to significantly reduce both systolic and diastolic blood pressure in individuals with hypertension.

Heart Health: By emphasizing whole, nutrient-dense foods and reducing the intake of saturated fats, red meat, and processed foods, the DASH Diet supports heart health. This, in turn, lowers the risk of heart disease, stroke, and other cardiovascular conditions.

Improved Cholesterol Levels: The diet's focus on lean proteins, whole grains, and a high intake of fruits and vegetables has been associated with improved cholesterol levels, particularly reducing LDL ("bad") cholesterol.

Weight Management: The DASH Diet, with its emphasis on whole foods and balanced nutrition, can aid in weight management. By promoting healthier food choices and balanced portions, it can help in maintaining a healthy weight.

Reduced Risk of Chronic Diseases: The DASH Diet's focus on whole foods, fruits, vegetables, and lean proteins has broader health implications. It's associated with a reduced risk of other chronic conditions, such as diabetes, certain cancers, and osteoporosis.

Improved Overall Nutrition: The diet encourages the consumption of nutrient-dense foods, ensuring a higher intake of essential vitamins, minerals, and antioxidants, supporting overall health and well-being.

Balanced Eating Patterns: The DASH Diet promotes balanced and healthy eating habits that are sustainable and adaptable. This can lead to long-term health benefits and overall better dietary habits.

Reduction in Sodium Intake: By lowering salt intake, the DASH Diet helps manage high blood pressure and decrease the risk of fluid retention, thereby aiding in the prevention of related health issues.

Promotion of Healthy Lifestyle Habits: It encourages not only dietary changes but also a healthier lifestyle, including increased physical activity and overall wellness.

Key Components and Food groups in the DASH Diet

Fruits:

- Aim for a variety of fruits, including berries, citrus fruits, apples, bananas, and others. They include essential vitamins, minerals, fiber, and antioxidants.

Vegetables:

- Encourages the consumption of various vegetables, both leafy greens and other colorful options. These offer vital nutrients, fiber, and antioxidants that contribute to good health.

Whole Grains:

- Incorporate whole grains such as brown rice, whole wheat, oats, quinoa, and whole-grain bread. They include fiber, B vitamins, and other important elements.

Lean Proteins:

- Choose lean protein sources like poultry (skinless), fish, beans, lentils, tofu, and nuts. These are lower in saturated fats and rich in nutrients like protein and healthy fats.

Low-Fat Dairy:

- Include low-fat or fat-free dairy products like milk, yogurt, and cheese to ensure an adequate intake of calcium and other essential nutrients.

Nuts, Seeds, and Legumes:

- These are excellent sources of protein, healthy fats, and various nutrients. Incorporate options like almonds, walnuts, flaxseeds, chia seeds, and beans into your diet.

Healthy Fats:

- Emphasize healthy fats from sources like olive oil, avocados, and nuts. These provide monounsaturated and polyunsaturated fats that support heart health.

Limited Saturated Fats and Added Sugars:

- The DASH Diet suggests reducing the intake of saturated fats found in red meat, processed foods, and full-fat dairy. Additionally, it advises limiting added sugars and sugary beverages.

Reduced Sodium Intake:

- To comply with the diet, it's important to decrease sodium consumption. This involves minimizing processed and high-sodium foods, using herbs and spices for flavor, and being mindful of salt intake.

Portion Control and Balanced Meals:

- Focus on balanced portion sizes and a variety of foods from these recommended groups to ensure a well-rounded diet.

Getting Started with the DASH Diet

Setting up your kitchen for success

Purge Unhealthy Options:

- Clear out your pantry, refrigerator, and freezer of processed and high-sodium foods, sugary snacks, and unhealthy fats. Donate or discard items that don't align with the DASH Diet.

Stock Up on Healthy Staples:

- Fill your kitchen with DASH-friendly foods like fresh fruits and vegetables, whole grains (brown rice, quinoa, whole-grain pasta), lean proteins (chicken, fish, beans), low-fat dairy, nuts, seeds, and healthy fats (olive oil, avocados).

Herbs, Spices, and Flavor Enhancers:

- Build a collection of herbs, spices, vinegar, and citrus to add flavor to your meals without relying on excessive salt. Options like garlic, pepper, basil, rosemary, and lemon juice can enhance the taste of your dishes.

Meal Prep Tools:

- Invest in tools that simplify healthy cooking, such as a good set of knives, cutting boards, steamer, non-stick pans, slow cooker, and food storage containers. These make meal preparation more efficient.

Label Reading and Shopping Skills:

- Familiarize yourself with reading food labels to identify high-sodium or processed items. Plan your grocery trips with a list of DASH-friendly foods to ensure you purchase the right items.

Meal Planning and Prepping:

- To make healthier choices, plan your meals ahead of time. Prepare a weekly meal plan and use it as a guide for grocery shopping and meal prep. Pre-cut vegetables, cook grains, and portion out snacks to save time during the week.

Organization and Accessibility:

- Organize your kitchen in a way that healthy options are easily accessible. Store fruits and cut vegetables at eye level in the refrigerator, keep whole grains and nuts in clear containers for easy visibility, and place unhealthy options out of sight.

Stay Hydrated:

- Have water readily available by keeping a reusable water bottle or jug within reach. Staying hydrated is an essential part of the DASH Diet and overall health.

Seek Inspiration and Resources:

- Utilize cookbooks, online resources, and apps that offer DASH-friendly recipes and meal plans. This can provide inspiration and support for your journey.

Grocery Shopping Tips and Essential Pantry Items

Grocery Shopping Tips:

- **Plan Ahead:** Make a list based on your weekly meal plan to avoid impulse purchases and ensure you have the necessary ingredients.

- **Shop the Perimeter:** Focus on fresh produce, lean proteins, and dairy located around the edges of the grocery store. These typically align with the DASH Diet principles.

- **Read Labels:** Check nutritional labels for sodium content, aiming for lower sodium options and avoiding high-sodium processed foods.

- **Choose Fresh Fruits and Vegetables:** Opt for a variety of colorful and seasonal fruits and vegetables, both fresh and frozen, to ensure you have a good mix.

- **Whole Grains:** Select whole grain options such as whole wheat bread, brown rice, quinoa, oats, and whole-grain pasta.

- **Lean Proteins:** Pick up lean protein sources like skinless poultry, fish, beans, lentils, tofu, and unsalted nuts.

- **Low-Fat Dairy:** Choose low-fat or fat-free dairy products like milk, yogurt, and cheese to meet calcium and protein needs.

- **Herbs, Spices, and Healthy Fats:** Purchase herbs, spices, olive oil, avocados, and nuts to add flavor and healthy fats to your meals.

Essential Pantry Items for the DASH Diet:

- **Whole Grains:** Brown rice, quinoa, whole-grain pasta, oats, whole-grain bread, and whole-grain cereals.

- **Canned Beans and Legumes:** Black beans, kidney beans, chickpeas, lentils, and other legumes, preferably with no added salt.

- **Canned or Dried Tomatoes:** A versatile ingredient for soups, stews, and sauces, but choose varieties without added salt or sugar.

- **Herbs and Spices:** Garlic powder, onion powder, cumin, turmeric, basil, oregano, pepper, paprika, and any other herbs and spices you enjoy.

- **Healthy Cooking Oils:** Olive oil, avocado oil, or other healthy oils for cooking and dressings.

- **Nuts and Seeds:** Almonds, walnuts, chia seeds, flaxseeds, and other unsalted nuts and seeds.

- **Low-Sodium Broth or Stock:** Use for soups and cooking to add flavor without excessive sodium.

- **Vinegar and Citrus:** Balsamic vinegar, apple cider vinegar, lemons, and limes for flavoring without adding salt.

Food to Include, Avoid or Limit in Dash Diet for Beginners

Foods to Include:

- **Fruits and Vegetables:** Aim for a variety of colorful fruits and vegetables rich in vitamins, minerals, and fiber.

- **Whole Grains:** Incorporate whole grains like brown rice, quinoa, whole wheat bread, and oats for fiber and nutrients.

- **Lean Proteins:** Include sources like poultry without skin, fish, beans, lentils, and nuts for protein.

- **Low-Fat Dairy:** Choose low-fat or fat-free options for milk, yogurt, and cheese to maintain calcium intake.

- **Healthy Fats:** Choose healthy fat sources such as olive oil, avocados, and almonds.

Foods to Limit:

- **Sodium:** Reduce intake of high-sodium foods like processed snacks, canned soups, and fast foods.

- **Sugary Foods:** Limit intake of sugary items such as soda, candies, and baked goods.

- **Red and Processed Meats:** Cut back on red meat and processed meats as they are higher in saturated fats.
- **Sweets and Desserts:** Limit desserts and sweets as they tend to be high in added sugars.

Foods to Avoid:

- **Highly Processed Foods:** Avoid highly processed, high-sodium, and high-sugar foods.
- **Trans Fats:** Stay away from foods high in trans fats which are typically found in many fried and baked goods.
- **Excessive Saturated Fats:** Limit foods high in saturated fats like full-fat dairy and fatty cuts of meat.

When starting the DASH Diet, beginners should focus on gradually introducing more fruits, vegetables, whole grains, lean proteins, and low-fat dairy while reducing sodium, added sugars, and unhealthy fats. It's essential to develop a balanced and sustainable approach to eating that aligns with the DASH Diet's principles for improved heart health and overall well-being.

Breakfast Recipes: Quick and Easy Breakfast Recipes

Greek Yogurt Parfait:

Ingredients:

- Low-fat Greek yogurt
- Fresh mixed berries (strawberries, blueberries, raspberries)
- Granola (low-sugar and low-sodium)
- Honey (optional)

Instructions:

- In a glass or bowl, layer Greek yogurt with mixed berries and granola.
- If desired, drizzle with honey for extra sweetness.
- Enjoy a protein-packed and flavorful breakfast.

Avocado Toast with Egg:

Ingredients:

- Whole-grain bread
- Ripe avocado
- Eggs

- Cherry tomatoes

- Salt and pepper

Instructions:

- Toast the whole-grain bread.

- Spread the mashed avocado on the toast.

- Cook an egg (poached, fried, or scrambled) and place it on top of the avocado.

- Add sliced cherry tomatoes, salt, and pepper to taste.

Berry Smoothie:

Ingredients:

- Mixed berries (strawberries, blueberries, raspberries)

- Low-fat Greek yogurt

- Unsweetened almond milk

- Spinach (optional)

- Chia seeds (optional)

Instructions:

- Blend mixed berries, a portion of Greek yogurt, a splash of almond milk, and spinach if desired.

- Add chia seeds for extra fiber and omega-3.

- Pour into a glass and enjoy a refreshing, nutrient-packed smoothie.

Oatmeal with Fruit and Nuts:

Ingredients:

- Rolled oats
- Water or unsweetened almond milk
- Sliced bananas or berries
- Chopped nuts (almonds, walnuts)
- Cinnamon (optional)

Instructions:

- Cook rolled oats with water or almond milk according to package instructions.
- Top with sliced bananas or berries and chopped nuts.
- Sprinkle with cinnamon for added flavor.

Egg and Vegetable Scramble:

Ingredients:

- Eggs
- Bell peppers (red, green, yellow)
- Spinach

- Onion

- Olive oil

- Salt and pepper

Instructions:

- Sauté diced bell peppers, onion, and spinach in a pan with a little olive oil.

- Whisk eggs, pour over the vegetables, and scramble until cooked.

- Season with salt and pepper.

Healthy and Nutritious Breakfast Options

Quinoa Breakfast Bowl:

Ingredients:

Cooked quinoa

- Low-fat Greek yogurt
- Sliced almonds or walnuts
- Mixed berries (blueberries, strawberries)
- Honey or a drizzle of maple syrup (optional)

Instructions:

- In a bowl, layer cooked quinoa with Greek yogurt.
- Top with mixed berries and sliced nuts.
- Drizzle with honey or maple syrup if desired for added sweetness.

Veggie Omelette:

Ingredients:

- Eggs
- Chopped vegetables (bell peppers, spinach, tomatoes)
- Low-fat feta cheese (optional)
- Olive oil
- Salt and pepper

Instructions:

- Sauté chopped vegetables in a pan with a little olive oil until tender.
- Whisk eggs, pour over the vegetables, and cook to make an omelette.
- Add a sprinkle of low-fat feta cheese if desired before folding the omelette.

Whole Grain Pancakes:

Ingredients:

- Whole-grain pancake mix or homemade batter
- Sliced bananas or blueberries
- Chopped nuts (pecans, almonds)
- Unsweetened applesauce (as a topping)

Instructions:

- Prepare pancakes using whole-grain mix or batter.

- Top with sliced bananas or blueberries and chopped nuts.

- Use unsweetened applesauce instead of syrup for a healthier option.

Smoked Salmon and Avocado Toast:

Ingredients:

- Whole-grain toast

- Smoked salmon

- Avocado slices

- Lemon juice

- Fresh dill (optional)

Instructions:

- Toast whole-grain bread.

- Spread avocado on the toast, top with smoked salmon.

- Squeeze a little lemon juice and garnish with fresh dill if desired.

Chia Seed Pudding:

Ingredients:

- Chia seeds
- Low-fat coconut milk or unsweetened almond milk
- Sliced mangoes or berries
- Shredded coconut (optional)

Instructions:

- Mix chia seeds and milk in a jar or bowl, let it sit overnight to form a pudding-like consistency.
- Top with sliced mangoes or berries and a sprinkle of shredded coconut.

Lunch Recipes: Delicious and Satisfying lunch Recipes

Mediterranean Chickpea Salad:

Ingredients:

- Canned chickpeas, rinsed and drained
- Diced cucumber, tomatoes, red onion
- Chopped fresh parsley and mint
- Kalamata olives (optional)
- Feta cheese (low-fat)
- Olive oil and lemon juice for dressing

Instructions:

- Combine chickpeas, diced vegetables, and herbs in a bowl.
- Add olives and crumbled feta cheese.
- To dress, drizzle with olive oil and lemon juice.

Grilled Chicken and Quinoa Bowl:

Ingredients:

- Grilled chicken breast, sliced

- Cooked quinoa

- Sliced bell peppers, zucchini, and red onion

- Spinach or mixed greens

- Balsamic vinaigrette (low-sodium)

Instructions:

- Grill the chicken and vegetables.

- Assemble a bowl with quinoa, grilled chicken, vegetables, and greens.

- Drizzle with balsamic vinaigrette.

Tuna and White Bean Salad:

Ingredients:

- Canned tuna in water, drained

- washed white beans (cannellini or navy)

- Celery, bell pepper, and onion, chopped

- Diced fresh parsley

- Sauce made with olive oil and red wine vinegar

Instructions:

- Combine tuna, white beans, chopped vegetables, and parsley in a bowl.

Toss with olive oil along with red wine vinegar until well combined.

Vegetarian Stuffed Bell Peppers:

Ingredients:

- Bell peppers, halved and deseeded

- Cooked quinoa or brown rice

- Black beans or lentils

- Chopped tomatoes, corn, and red onion

- Shredded low-fat cheese (optional)

Instructions:

- Preheat the oven. Mix cooked quinoa, beans, vegetables, and spices in a bowl.

- Stuff the pepper halves with the mixture and bake until peppers are tender.

- Top with shredded cheese if desired.

Whole Grain Wrap with Hummus and Veggies:

Ingredients:

- Whole grain wrap or tortilla
- Hummus (low-sodium)
- Sliced cucumbers, shredded carrots, mixed greens
- Sliced avocado (optional)

Instructions:

- Spread hummus on the wrap.
- Layer with sliced vegetables and avocado.
- Roll up the wrap and slice in half.

Variations for Different Tastes and Dietary Needs

Vegetarian or Vegan Options:

- Substitute animal proteins with plant-based alternatives like tofu, tempeh, or seitan in recipes that call for chicken or tuna.
- Opt for plant-based cheese or omit cheese entirely for vegan options.
- Use plant-based protein sources such as beans, lentils, or chickpeas in place of meat in salads or bowls.

Gluten-Free Adaptations:

- Replace wheat-based ingredients with gluten-free options like quinoa, brown rice, or gluten-free pasta in grain-based dishes.
- Ensure salad dressings and marinades are gluten-free or make your own using gluten-free ingredients.
- Use gluten-free wraps or lettuce leaves in place of wheat-based wraps for sandwiches or wraps.

Low-Sodium Variations:

- Rinse canned beans or vegetables thoroughly to reduce sodium content.

- Avoid or reduce the use of high-sodium ingredients like olives or certain canned products.

- Opt for fresh herbs, spices, and vinegar to add flavor instead of salt in dressings or marinades.

Low-Fat Options:

- Choose low-fat or fat-free dairy options in recipes that call for cheese or yogurt.

- Use less oil when sautéing vegetables or grilling proteins.

- For salads or bowls, limit the use of high-fat dressings and opt for lighter vinaigrettes or homemade dressings with less oil.

Allergies or Specific Dietary Restrictions:

- Swap nuts for seeds or omit them entirely for nut allergies.

- Check for individual allergies and sensitivities and make appropriate substitutions. For instance, use sunflower seed butter instead of peanut butter.

- Adjust ingredients to accommodate specific dietary requirements, such as keto, paleo, or other specialized diets, if necessary.

Customized Seasonings and Flavors:

- Tailor spices and seasonings to suit personal taste preferences.

- Experiment with various herbs and spices to add unique flavors without compromising the DASH Diet guidelines.

- Consider adding a touch of heat with chili flakes or hot sauce for those who enjoy spicier flavors.

Dinner Recipes: Flavorful and Balanced Dinner Options

Baked Lemon Herb Salmon:

Ingredients:

- Salmon fillets
- Fresh lemon juice
- Chopped fresh dill, parsley, and garlic
- Olive oil
- Salt and pepper

Instructions:

- Preheat the oven. Place salmon on a baking sheet.
- Mix lemon juice, herbs, garlic, and olive oil. Brush over the salmon.
- Bake the salmon until it is cooked through and readily flakes.

Mediterranean Vegetable and Chickpea Stew:

Ingredients:

- Diced eggplant, zucchini, bell peppers
- Chickpeas (canned, rinsed)
- Chopped tomatoes or tomato sauce
- Chopped onion and garlic
- Fresh basil and oregano
- Olive oil

Instructions:

- In olive oil, sauté the onion and garlic until tender.
- Add chopped vegetables.
- Stir in tomatoes, chickpeas, and herbs. Simmer until the vegetables are tender.

Grilled Chicken with Quinoa and Roasted Vegetables:

Ingredients:

- Grilled chicken breast
- Cooked quinoa

- Vegetables that have been roasted (such as broccoli, carrots, and bell peppers)
- Olive oil, garlic, and herbs for roasting

Instructions:

- Roast vegetables with olive oil, garlic, and herbs until tender.
- Serve grilled chicken with quinoa and the roasted vegetables.

Turkey and Black Bean Tacos:

Ingredients:

- Ground turkey
- Black beans (canned, rinsed)
- Taco seasoning (low-sodium)
- Whole-grain tortillas
- Toppings: Shredded lettuce, diced tomatoes, salsa, and low-fat Greek yogurt

Instructions:

- Cook ground turkey with taco seasoning. Add black beans.
- Serve the turkey and bean mixture in whole-grain tortillas with desired toppings.

Vegetarian Stir-Fry with Tofu:

Ingredients:

- Cubed tofu

- Mixed stir-fry vegetables (bell peppers, broccoli, snap peas)

- Soy sauce (low-sodium)

- Sesame oil

- Garlic and ginger

Instructions:

- Sauté tofu until golden. Add mixed vegetables, garlic, and ginger.

- Stir in soy sauce and sesame oil. Cook until vegetables are tender-crisp.

One-Pot Meals, Quick Recipes, and Family-Friendly Dinners

One-Pot Chicken and Brown Rice:

Ingredients:

- Chicken thighs or breasts
- Brown rice
- Chopped onions, bell peppers, and garlic
- Low-sodium chicken broth
- Herbs (like thyme, rosemary)

Instructions:

- Brown chicken in a pot. Cook until the vegetables are soft.
- Stir in brown rice, herbs, and chicken broth. Simmer until rice is cooked and chicken is tender.

Vegetable and White Bean Soup:

Ingredients:

- Mixed vegetables (carrots, celery, zucchini)
- Canned white beans (cannellini or navy beans)
- Low-sodium vegetable broth

- Chopped onions and garlic

- Herbs (such as basil, oregano)

Instructions:

- Sauté onions and garlic, add mixed vegetables and beans.

- Pour in vegetable broth, add herbs, and simmer until vegetables are tender.

Pasta Primavera with Shrimp:

Ingredients:

- Whole-grain pasta

- Shrimp

- Mixed vegetables (zucchini, cherry tomatoes, bell peppers)

- Olive oil, garlic, and lemon juice

Instructions:

- Cook pasta according to package directions.

- Sauté shrimp and vegetables in olive oil and garlic. Toss with cooked pasta and lemon juice.

Quick and Easy Beef Stir-Fry:

Ingredients:

- Lean beef strips

- Stir-fry vegetables (broccoli, snow peas, carrots)

- Low-sodium soy sauce

- Garlic and ginger

- Brown rice or quinoa

Instructions:

- Stir-fry beef until browned, add vegetables, garlic, and ginger.

- Pour in soy sauce, cook until the vegetables are tender-crisp. Serve with brown rice or quinoa.

Sheet Pan Baked Fish and Vegetables:

Ingredients:

- Fillets of white fish (such as either cod or tilapia)

- Sliced bell peppers, asparagus, and cherry tomatoes

- Olive oil, lemon juice, and herbs

Instructions:

- Preheat oven. Place fish on a baking sheet, surround with vegetables.

- Drizzle with olive oil, lemon juice, and herbs. Bake until fish is cooked and vegetables are tender.

Snacks and Sides: Nutritious Snack Ideas and Side Dishes

Nutritious Snack Ideas:

Vegetable Sticks with Hummus:

- Sliced cucumbers, bell peppers, and carrots served with a portion of low-sodium hummus.

Greek Yogurt with Berries:

- Low-fat Greek yogurt topped with fresh berries (blueberries, strawberries, raspberries).

Homemade Trail Mix:

- Mix unsalted nuts (almonds, walnuts) with dried fruits (apricots, cranberries) and a few dark chocolate pieces.

Apple Slices with Nut Butter:

- Apple slices paired with a tablespoon of natural nut or seed butter (almond, peanut, or sunflower seed butter).

Rice Cakes with Avocado:

Brown rice cakes topped with mashed avocado and a sprinkle of black pepper or a dash of hot sauce.

Whole Grain Crackers with Cottage Cheese:

Whole grain crackers served with low-fat cottage cheese and sliced tomatoes or cucumber.

Nutritious Side Dishes:

Quinoa Salad:

- A cold salad made with cooked quinoa, mixed with diced vegetables, such as cucumber, bell peppers, and cherry tomatoes, dressed with lemon juice and olive oil.

Steamed Vegetables:

- Lightly steamed mixed vegetables such as broccoli, cauliflower, and carrots seasoned with herbs like parsley, thyme, and a hint of olive oil.

Mixed Bean Salad:

- A medley of beans (black beans, kidney beans, cannellini beans) mixed with chopped red onions, bell peppers, and a light vinaigrette.

Whole Grain Bread with Olive Oil and Herbs:

- Slices of whole grain bread served with a side of extra virgin olive oil mixed with garlic, herbs, and a sprinkle of Parmesan cheese.

Cucumber Tomato Salad:

- Sliced cucumbers and cherry tomatoes tossed with red onion, fresh herbs, a drizzle of balsamic vinegar, and a touch of olive oil.

Brown Rice or Quinoa Pilaf:

- Cooked brown rice or quinoa mixed with sautéed onions, garlic, and mixed vegetables, flavored with a squeeze of lemon juice.

Dips, salads, and small bites

Dips:

- **Guacamole:** Mashed avocado mixed with diced tomatoes, onions, cilantro, lime juice, and a touch of salt. Serve with vegetable sticks or whole grain pita chips.

- **White Bean Dip:** Blend white beans, garlic, lemon juice, and fresh herbs like rosemary or thyme. Serve with whole grain crackers or vegetables, if desired.

- **Tzatziki:** Greek yogurt mixed with grated cucumber, minced garlic, dill, and a splash of lemon juice. Ideal for dipping fresh vegetable sticks or whole wheat pita triangles.

Salads:

- **Kale and Quinoa Salad:** Raw kale massaged with olive oil and lemon juice, mixed with cooked quinoa, cherry tomatoes, sliced almonds, and a sprinkle of feta cheese.

- **Mediterranean Orzo Salad:** Orzo pasta mixed with diced cucumbers, cherry tomatoes, Kalamata olives, red onions, parsley, and dressed with olive oil and red wine vinegar.

- **Spinach and Strawberry Salad:** Fresh spinach leaves with sliced strawberries, crumbled feta cheese, and walnuts. Drizzle with a light vinaigrette made of balsamic vinegar and a touch of olive oil.

Small Bites:

- **Stuffed Mushrooms:** Mushroom caps filled with a mixture of breadcrumbs, chopped spinach, garlic, and a touch of Parmesan cheese, then baked until golden.

- **Caprese Skewers:** Alternate cherry tomatoes, fresh mozzarella balls, and basil leaves on small skewers. Drizzle with a touch of balsamic glaze.

- **Turkey and Veggie Lettuce Wraps:** Lettuce leaves filled with lean turkey slices, shredded carrots, cucumbers, and a dollop of hummus or tzatziki

Desserts and Treats: Healthier Dessert Alternatives

Fruit Salad with Yogurt:

- A refreshing mix of assorted fresh fruits such as berries, melons, and citrus segments served with a dollop of low-fat Greek yogurt and a sprinkle of chopped nuts.

Dark Chocolate-Dipped Strawberries:

- Fresh strawberries dipped in melted dark chocolate (70% cocoa or higher). Let them cool and harden on a parchment-lined tray for a delightful treat.

Frozen Banana Bites:

- Sliced bananas dipped in a thin layer of melted dark chocolate and topped with chopped nuts, then frozen until solid.

Greek Yogurt Parfait:

- Layer low-fat Greek yogurt with fresh fruits, a drizzle of honey, and a sprinkle of granola or crushed nuts for added texture and flavor.

Baked Apples:

- Apples cored and filled with a mixture of oats, cinnamon, a touch of honey or maple syrup, then baked until tender. Serve with a dollop of Greek yogurt or a sprinkle of nuts.

Chia Seed Pudding with Berries:

- Chia seeds soaked in unsweetened almond milk or low-fat coconut milk, sweetened with a touch of honey or pureed berries. Serve with fresh berries on top.

Homemade Fruit Sorbet:

- Blend frozen mixed berries or mango chunks with a touch of honey or agave syrup until smooth and creamy. Serve as a refreshing sorbet.

Coconut Date Rolls:

- Combine dates, shredded coconut, and a touch of cocoa powder in a food processor. Roll the mixture into small balls and coat with additional coconut.

Yogurt-Covered Frozen Grapes:

- Dip grapes in low-fat yogurt and freeze until the yogurt hardens, creating a sweet and refreshing snack.

Moderation and Sweet treats Aligned with the DASH Diet

Dark Chocolate:

- Opt for high-quality dark chocolate (70% cocoa or higher) in moderation. Enjoy a couple of squares as a treat. Dark chocolate contains antioxidants and lower sugar content compared to milk chocolate.

Fruit-Based Sorbets:

- Make homemade sorbets using pureed fruits with minimal added sugar or opt for store-bought varieties with no added sugars or artificial sweeteners.

Homemade Fruit Popsicles:

- Blend pureed fruits like berries, mango, or pineapple with a bit of natural sweetener (if needed) and freeze in popsicle molds for a refreshing and healthier sweet treat.

Natural Fruit Bars:

- Choose frozen fruit bars made with 100% real fruit and no added sugars, or make your own by freezing pureed fruits.

Yogurt and Fruit Parfaits:

- Layer low-fat yogurt with fresh fruits, a drizzle of honey or a small amount of granola for crunch in small portions.

Baked Treats with Reduced Sugar:

- Experiment with baking by reducing the sugar content in recipes for muffins, cookies, or cakes. Substitute with natural sweeteners like applesauce, mashed bananas, or dates.

Fruit and Nut Trail Mix:

- Create your own trail mix with a mix of unsalted nuts, dried fruits like apricots, raisins, and a small amount of dark chocolate chips for a sweet touch.

Healthy Energy Balls:

- Make energy balls using a combination of nuts, dates, oats, and a touch of cocoa for a natural and sweet energy-boosting treat.

Low-Sugar Baked Fruit Desserts:

- Explore recipes for baked apples, pears, or peaches with minimal added sugar, enhanced with spices like cinnamon or nutmeg.

Quick and Easy Recipes for Busy Days

Mediterranean Chickpea Salad:

Ingredients:

- Canned chickpeas, drained and rinsed
- Diced cucumber, cherry tomatoes, red onion
- Chopped fresh parsley and mint
- Feta cheese (low-fat)
- Olive oil, lemon juice, salt, and pepper

Instructions:

- In a mixing dish, mix all of the ingredients.
- Garnish with pepper and salt to taste and drizzle using olive oil along with lemon juice.
- Toss and serve.

Veggie Omelette:

Ingredients:

- Eggs
- Chopped vegetables (bell peppers, spinach, tomatoes)
- Olive oil, salt, and pepper

Instructions:

- Sauté vegetables in a pan with olive oil.
- Beat eggs, pour over the vegetables. Cook until set. Add salt and pepper to taste.

Tuna and White Bean Salad:

Ingredients:

- Canned tuna in water, drained
- washed white beans either cannellini or navy beans)
- Celery, red bell pepper, and red onion, chopped
- Red wine vinegar, olive oil, pepper, and salt to taste

Instructions:

- Combine all ingredients in a bowl.
- Dress with Red wine vinegar, olive oil, pepper, and salt to taste. Mix well and serve.

Whole Grain Wrap with Hummus and Veggies:

Ingredients:

- Whole grain wrap or tortilla
- Hummus (low-sodium)
- Sliced cucumbers, shredded carrots, mixed greens

Instructions:

- Spread hummus on the wrap.
- Layer with sliced vegetables and mixed greens. Roll and serve.

Pasta Primavera with Grilled Chicken:

Ingredients:

- Whole-grain pasta
- Grilled chicken breast, sliced
- Vegetables (bell peppers, zucchini, and cherry tomatoes)
- Olive oil, garlic, salt, and pepper

Instructions:

- Cook pasta according to package directions.
- Sauté vegetables in olive oil and garlic. Toss with pasta and grilled chicken. Season with salt and pepper.

Recipes for Specific Dietary Needs (e.g., vegetarian, gluten-free)

Vegetarian Recipes:

Vegetarian Chili:

Ingredients:

- Mixed beans (kidney beans, black beans, pinto beans)
- Diced tomatoes
- Chopped bell peppers, onions, and garlic
- Vegetable broth
- Chili powder, cumin, paprika

Instructions:

- Sauté vegetables in a pot, add beans, diced tomatoes, spices, and broth.
- Simmer until flavors meld and the chili thickens.

Eggplant and Chickpea Curry:

Ingredients:

- Diced eggplant
- Cooked chickpeas
- Chopped tomatoes, onions, garlic, and ginger
- Curry spices (turmeric, cumin, coriander)

Instructions:

- Sauté onions, garlic, and spices. Add eggplant, chickpeas, and tomatoes.
- Simmer until the eggplant is tender.

Gluten-Free Recipes:

Quinoa Stuffed Bell Peppers:

Ingredients:

- Bell peppers, halved and deseeded
- Cooked quinoa
- Black beans, corn, diced tomatoes
- Shredded cheese (optional)

Instructions:

- Combine cooked quinoa, black beans, corn, tomatoes, and seasonings in a mixing bowl. Stuff into pepper halves.
- Bake until peppers are tender. Sprinkle with cheese if desired.

Grilled Lemon Herb Chicken with Roasted Vegetables:

Ingredients:

- Grilled chicken breast
- Assorted vegetables (zucchini, bell peppers, broccoli)
- Olive oil, garlic, lemon juice, herbs

Instructions:

- Toss vegetables in olive oil, garlic, and herbs. Roast until tender.
- Serve with grilled chicken marinated in lemon juice and herbs.

Tips for Dining out and Sticking to the DASH Diet

1. **Plan Ahead:**

   - Check the restaurant's menu online before going. Many restaurants now provide their menus on their websites, allowing you to make more informed choices in advance.

2. **Look for Healthy Options:**

   - Seek out dishes that contain a variety of vegetables, whole grains, and lean proteins. Opt for salads, grilled or steamed options, and meals with minimal added sauces or dressings.

3. **Ask Questions:**

   - Don't hesitate to ask the server about the preparation or ingredients of a dish. Request substitutions or modifications to suit your dietary preferences.

4. **Control Portions:**

   - Restaurant portions are frequently bigger than necessary. Consider sharing an entrée, or ask for a to-go box at the start and pack up half your meal to eat later.

5. Choose Grilled or Steamed:

- Select items that are grilled, steamed, or baked rather than fried. These cooking methods are usually lower in added fats and oils.

6. Be Mindful of Sauces and Dressings:

- Request sauces and dressings on the side. Use them sparingly to control the amount of added salt, sugar, and fat in your meal.

7. Avoid or Limit Extras:

- Steer clear of high-calorie extras like bread baskets, appetizers, or desserts, or limit them to one healthier choice.

8. Watch Your Salt Intake:

- Ask for dishes with minimal salt or request that your meal be prepared without added salt, as excess sodium can be an issue in restaurant food.

9. Consider Beverages:

- Drink unsweetened tea, water, or other drinks with fewer calories instead.

- Avoid sugary drinks and alcoholic beverages, which can add unnecessary calories and sugar.

10. Practice Moderation:

- Enjoy your meal mindfully. Take your time eating, savor the flavors, and stop when you feel satisfied. Listen to your body's signals of fullness.

Lifestyle and Long-Term Success

- **Gradual Changes:** Implement changes gradually. Begin by include more fruits, veggies, and whole grains in your diet. Slowly reduce the intake of processed foods, sodium, and added sugars.

- **Regular Physical Activity:** Alongside a healthy diet, regular exercise is crucial for overall well-being. Aim for at least 150 minutes of moderate aerobic activity per week, such as brisk walking, or follow guidelines provided by your healthcare professional.

- **Meal Planning:** Plan your meals in advance. This helps in making healthier food choices, controlling portions, and reducing reliance on convenience or fast food.

- **Portion Control:** Be mindful of portion sizes. Using smaller plates, dividing leftovers for future meals, and being aware of appropriate serving sizes can help manage caloric intake.

- **Balanced Diet:** Ensure meals are balanced with a variety of nutrient-dense foods, including fruits, vegetables, lean proteins, whole grains, and healthy fats. This helps meet nutritional needs and supports long-term health.

- **Drink enough of water all through the day to keep yourself hydrated.**

- Water helps maintain proper bodily functions and aids in controlling appetite.

- **Stress Management:** Manage stress through techniques like meditation, yoga, or hobbies. Stress can have an impact on eating habits and general health.

- **Seek Support:** Consider seeking guidance from a registered dietitian or nutritionist who can provide personalized advice, making it easier to adhere to the DASH Diet long-term.

- **Accountability and Tracking:** Keep a food diary to track your intake. This helps in recognizing patterns, making adjustments, and staying accountable for your choices.

- **Flexibility:** Be flexible. While striving to follow the DASH Diet, allow yourself occasional treats or deviations. Long-term success is about finding a sustainable balance.

- **Regular Check-ups:** Regularly monitor your blood pressure and overall health. Consult healthcare professionals for advice and guidance on your dietary needs.

Nutritional Information

Nutritional Information of Common Foods:

PLEASE NOTE: Nutritional content can vary based on brand, preparation, and serving sizes.

1. **Fruits and Vegetables:**

   - Most fruits and vegetables are low in fat and calories but high in vitamins, minerals, and fiber.

   - For specific nutritional information, you can refer to USDA's National Nutrient Database or similar resources.

2. **Proteins:**

   - Chicken breast (skinless, cooked) provides protein with low fat content.

   - Fish like salmon is high in protein and healthy fats like omega-3 fatty acids.

   - Protein and fiber are abundant in legumes such as lentils and chickpeas.

3. **Grains:**

- Whole grains like brown rice, quinoa, and whole wheat pasta offer fiber and essential nutrients.

4. **Dairy and Alternatives:**

- Low-fat dairy products provide calcium and protein.

- Plant-based alternatives like almond milk or soy milk can be fortified with nutrients such as calcium and vitamin D.

Nutritional Table Chart

Food Item	Carbohydrates (g)	Protein (g)	Fat (g)	Calories	Micronutrients
Spinach (1 cup, cooked)	7	5	1	41	Iron, Vitamin K, Vitamin A
Salmon (3 oz)	0	20	7	175	Omega-3 Fatty Acids, Vitamin D, Vitamin B12
Brown Rice (1 cup)	45	5	1	216	Magnesium, Phosphorus, B Vitamins
Greek Yogurt (6 oz)	7	17	0.7	100	Calcium, Probiotics, Vitamin D
Chickpeas (1 cup, canned)	45	12	4	269	Fiber, Potassium, Iron
Berries (1 cup)	15	1	0.5	60	Vitamin C, Fiber, Antioxidants
Quinoa (1 cup, cooked)	39	8	4	222	Iron, Magnesium, Fiber

Food Item	Carbohydrates (g)	Protein (g)	Fat (g)	Calories	Micronutrients
Chicken Breast (3 oz)	0	26	3	142	Protein, Vitamin B6, Selenium
Almonds (1 oz)	6	6	14	160	Vitamin E, Magnesium, Healthy Fats
Sweet Potatoes (1 medium)	26	2	0.2	103	Vitamin A, Vitamin C, Potassium

BONUS

30 Days Meal Plan

Day	Breakfast	Lunch	Dinner
1	Greek yogurt with mixed berries and almonds	Quinoa salad with chickpeas, tomatoes, cucumbers	Baked salmon, lemon-dill, steamed broccoli, brown rice
2	Whole grain toast with avocado and poached eggs	Lentil soup with mixed green salad	Grilled chicken, roasted sweet potatoes, sautéed spinach
3	Oatmeal with sliced bananas and Greek yogurt	Whole wheat wrap with hummus, veggies, grilled shrimp	Vegetable stir-fry with tofu over quinoa
4	Berry and banana smoothie with protein powder	Turkey and vegetable whole grain wrap, sliced apples	Whole wheat pasta with marinara, grilled chicken, steamed green beans
5	Scrambled eggs with sautéed mushrooms, tomatoes, whole grain	Spinach and feta-stuffed chicken, quinoa,	Baked cod with citrus glaze, brown rice, side

Day	Breakfast	Lunch	Dinner
	toast	steamed asparagus	salad
6	Cottage cheese with sliced peaches, handful of walnuts	Black bean and vegetable burrito bowl, brown rice	Stir-fried shrimp, broccoli, brown rice
7	Whole grain waffles with fresh berries, honey	Mediterranean chickpea salad with diced tomatoes, cucumber, olives	Grilled vegetable and quinoa-stuffed bell peppers
8	Whole grain bagel with smoked salmon, cream cheese, sliced tomatoes	Quinoa and black bean bowl with salsa, avocado	Grilled turkey burgers, whole wheat buns, lettuce, tomato, oven-baked sweet potato fries
9	Berry and spinach smoothie with protein powder	Lentil and vegetable soup, whole grain crackers	Baked cod with citrus glaze, quinoa, steamed asparagus
10	Greek yogurt parfait with granola, mixed berries	Spinach and feta-stuffed mushrooms, brown rice	Baked chicken breast, balsamic glaze, quinoa, roasted Brussels

Day	Breakfast	Lunch	Dinner
			sprouts
11	Whole grain waffles with fruit compote, Greek yogurt	Turkey and vegetable whole wheat wrap, sliced cucumbers	Grilled shrimp skewers, mango salsa, brown rice, steamed broccoli
12	Scrambled eggs with sautéed mushrooms, spinach, whole grain toast	Mediterranean quinoa salad, cherry tomatoes, cucumber, olives	Baked eggplant parmesan, mixed green salad
13	Avocado and tomato toast on whole grain bread	Overnight oats with diced apples, cinnamon	Stir-fried tofu, broccoli, bell peppers, brown rice
14	Oatmeal with sliced bananas, walnuts, honey	Spinach and feta-stuffed chicken, quinoa, steamed broccoli	Shrimp and vegetable skewers, quinoa
15	Whole grain pancakes with fresh berries, almonds	Tuna salad with mixed greens, cherry tomatoes, cucumber	Baked salmon, lemon and dill, quinoa, steamed asparagus
16	Berry and spinach smoothie with protein	Lentil and vegetable soup, whole grain	Stir-fried tofu, broccoli, bell peppers, brown

Day	Breakfast	Lunch	Dinner
	powder	crackers	rice
17	Greek yogurt parfait with granola, mixed berries	Spinach and feta-stuffed chicken, quinoa, steamed broccoli	Baked chicken breast, balsamic glaze, quinoa, roasted Brussels sprouts
18	Whole grain waffles with fruit compote, Greek yogurt	Turkey and vegetable whole wheat wrap, sliced cucumbers	Grilled shrimp skewers, mango salsa, brown rice, steamed broccoli
19	Scrambled eggs with sautéed mushrooms, spinach, whole grain toast	Mediterranean quinoa salad, cherry tomatoes, cucumber, olives	Baked eggplant parmesan, mixed green salad
20	Avocado and tomato toast on whole grain bread	Overnight oats with diced apples, cinnamon	Stir-fried tofu, broccoli, bell peppers, brown rice
21	Oatmeal with sliced bananas, walnuts, honey	Caprese salad with grilled chicken breast	Grilled vegetable and quinoa-stuffed bell peppers

Day	Breakfast	Lunch	Dinner
22	Whole grain bagel with smoked salmon, cream cheese, sliced tomatoes	Quinoa and black bean bowl with salsa, avocado	Grilled turkey burgers, whole wheat buns, lettuce, tomato, oven-baked sweet potato fries
23	Berry and spinach smoothie with protein powder	Lentil and vegetable soup, whole grain crackers	Baked cod with citrus glaze, quinoa, steamed asparagus
24	Greek yogurt parfait with granola, mixed berries	Spinach and feta-stuffed chicken, quinoa, steamed broccoli	Stir-fried tofu, broccoli, bell peppers, brown rice
25	Whole grain waffles with fruit compote, Greek yogurt	Turkey and vegetable whole wheat wrap, sliced cucumbers	Baked chicken breast, balsamic glaze, quinoa, roasted Brussels sprouts
26	Scrambled eggs with sautéed mushrooms, spinach, whole grain toast	Mediterranean quinoa salad, cherry tomatoes, cucumber, olives	Grilled shrimp skewers, mango salsa, brown rice, steamed broccoli

Day	Breakfast	Lunch	Dinner
27	Avocado and tomato toast on whole grain bread	Chicken and vegetable stir-fry, brown rice	Vegetable and lentil curry, basmati rice
28	Oatmeal with sliced bananas, walnuts, honey	Caprese salad with grilled chicken breast	Baked eggplant lasagna, mixed green salad
29	Whole grain pancakes with fresh berries, almonds	Tuna salad with mixed greens, cherry tomatoes, cucumber	Baked salmon, lemon and dill, quinoa, steamed asparagus
30	Berry and spinach smoothie with protein powder	Greek-inspired chicken wrap, whole wheat tortilla	Grilled vegetable and quinoa-stuffed bell peppers